Healthful lifestyle: Rapid healthiness to get a healthy life to produce a positive outcome.

John.O.Dennis

Table of content

Introduction

When you're not at your healthiest, you can probably tell. You may simply feel "off." You may find that you feel tired, your digestive system isn't functioning as well as it normally does, and you seem to catch colds. Mentally, you may find you can't focus and feel nervous or sad.

The good news: a healthy lifestyle may help you feel better. Even better, you don't have to redesign your whole life overnight. It's quite simple to make a couple of tiny modifications that may lead you in the direction of increased well-being. And after you make one adjustment, that success might drive you to continue to make other beneficial improvements.

What is a "healthy lifestyle"? Ask 50 individuals to explain what a "healthy lifestyle" is, and you'll likely receive 50 different replies. That's because there's no one way to be healthy. A healthy lifestyle simply involves doing activities that make you happy and feel well.

For one individual, it may mean walking a mile five times a week, eating fast food once a week, and spending virtual or in-person time with loved ones every other day. For someone else, a healthy lifestyle may involve training and running two marathons a year, following a keto diet, and never drinking a taste of alcohol.

Neither of these is better than the other. Both are excellent for that individual. You get to select what your healthy lifestyle looks like.

Chapter 1

Eating Nutritious Meals To Enhance The Body's Immune System

The key to a healthy diet is to eat the right amount of calories for how active you are, so you balance the energy you consume with the energy you use.

If you eat or drink more than your body requires, you'll put on weight because the energy you do not utilize is stored as fat. If you eat and drink too little, you'll lose weight.

You should also consume a broad selection of foods to make sure you're getting a balanced diet and your body is obtaining all the nutrients it needs.

It's advised that males consume roughly 2,500 calories a day (10,500 kilojoules) (10,500 kilojoules). Women should consume roughly 2,000 calories a day (8,400 kilojoules) (eight thousand kilojoules).

Most people in the UK are consuming more calories than they require and should consume fewer calories.

1.Base your meals on higher-fiber starchy carbs. Starchy carbs should make up a little over a third of the meals you consume. They include potatoes, bread, rice, pasta, and cereals.

Choose higher fiber or wholegrain options, such as wholewheat pasta, brown rice or potatoes with their skins on.

They include more fiber than white or refined starchy carbs and might help you feel full for longer.

Try to incorporate at least 1 starchy item with each main meal. Some people assume starchy meals are fattening, although gram for gram, the carbohydrates they contain deliver less than half the calories of fat.

Keep an eye on the fats you add while you're preparing or serving these sorts of meals since that's what raises the calorie count-for example, oil on chips, butter on toast, and creamy sauces on pasta.

2. Eat plenty of fruit and vegetables. It's advised that you consume at least 5 pieces of a variety of fruit and vegetables every day. They may be fresh, frozen, tinned, dried, or juiced.

3. Consume more fish, particularly fatty fish.Fish is a rich source of protein and includes numerous vitamins and minerals.
Aim to consume at least 2 servings of fish a week, including at least 1 meal of oily fish.
Oily fish are abundant in omega-3 lipids, which may help prevent heart disease.

Oily fish include:
•salmons
•trouts
•herrings
•sardines
•pilchards
•mackerel

Non-oily fish include:
•haddocks
•plaices
•coleys
•cods
•tunas
•skates
•hake

You may select from fresh, frozen, and canned fish, but note that canned and smoked fish can be rich in salt.
Most individuals should be eating more fish, but there are advised limitations for particular species of fish.

4. Cut down on saturated fat and sugar. 5. Saturated fat You need some fat in your diet, but it's crucial to pay attention to the quantity and kind of fat you're consuming. There are two basic forms of fat: saturated and unsaturated. Too much saturated fat may raise the quantity of cholesterol in the

blood, which increases your chance of getting heart disease.

On average, males should consume no more than 30g of saturated fat a day. On average, women should eat no more than 20g of saturated fat a day.

Children under the age of 11 should have less saturated fat than adults, but a low-fat diet is not suited for children under 5.

Saturated fat is present in numerous foods, such as:

•fatty meat pieces•sausages•butters•hard cheeses•creams•cakes•biscuits•lards•pies

Try to cut down on your saturated fat consumption and pick foods that contain unsaturated fats instead, such as vegetable oils and spreads, oily salmon, and avocados.

For a healthy alternative, use a tiny quantity of vegetable or olive oil, or reduced-fat spread instead of butter, lard or ghee.

When you're consuming meat, choose lean cuts and chop off any visible fat.

All forms of fat are rich in energy, hence they should only be taken in tiny quantities.

Regularly eating meals and beverages rich in sugar raises your chances of obesity and tooth disease.

Sugary meals and beverages are generally rich in energy (measured in kilojoules or calories) and, if taken too regularly, may lead to weight gain. They may also promote tooth decay, particularly if consumed between meals.

Free sugars are any sugars added to meals or beverages, or found naturally in honey, syrups, and unsweetened fruit juices and smoothies.

This is the sort of sugar you should be cutting down on, rather than the sugar found in fruit and milk.

Many packaged meals and beverages contain shockingly large quantities of free sugar.

Free sugars are present in numerous foods, such as:

•Sugary fizzy drinks

•Sugary breakfast cereals
•Cakes
•Biscuits
•Pastries and puddings
•Sweets and chocolates
•Alcoholic beverages

5. Limit your salt intake to no more than 6g per day for adults.Eating too much salt might increase your blood pressure. People with high blood pressure are more prone to developing heart disease or having a stroke.
Even if you do not add salt to your dishes, you may still be consuming too much.
About three-quarters of the salt you consume is already in the product when you purchase it, such as morning cereals, soups, breads, and sauces.

6. Be physically active and maintain a healthy weight.As well as eating correctly, frequent exercise may help minimize your chance of having major health disorders. It's

also vital for your general health and wellness.

Being overweight or obese may lead to health issues such as type 2 diabetes, some malignancies, heart disease, and stroke. Being underweight might also harm your health.

Most individuals need to lose weight by consuming fewer calories.

If you're wanting to lose weight, strive to eat less and be more active. Eating a healthy, balanced diet may help you maintain a healthy weight.

Do not become thirsty. You need to consume lots of fluids to avoid becoming dehydrated. The government suggests drinking 6 to 8 cups per day. This is in addition to the fluid you acquire from the food you consume.

All non-alcoholic beverages qualify, although water, reduced fat milk, and lower sugar drinks, including tea and coffee, are better alternatives.

Try to avoid sugary soft and fizzy beverages since they're high in calories. They're also terrible for your teeth.

Even unsweetened fruit juice and smoothies are rich in free sugar.

Your combined amount of beverages from fruit juice, vegetable juice, and smoothies should not be more than 150ml a day, which is a tiny glass.

Remember to consume extra water during hot weather or when exercising.

Do not miss breakfast. Some folks skip breakfast because they believe it'll help them lose weight.

But a nutritious breakfast rich in fibre and low in fat, sugar and salt may form part of a balanced diet and can help you obtain the nutrients you need for optimal health.

A wholegrain reduced sugar cereal with semi-skimmed milk and fruit cut over the top is a great and healthy meal.

Chapter 2

Make A Suitable Choice On A Health Path.

Using a step-by-step decision-making process will help you make more deliberate and meaningful judgments by organizing important information and clarifying options. This strategy enhances the likelihood that you will select the most pleasing choice possible.

Steps include the following:

•Step 1: Determine the decisionYou know that you need to make a choice. Try to clearly identify the essence of the choice you must make. This initial step is really crucial.

•Step 2: Gather the required informationCollect some essential information before you make your decision: what information is required, the best sources of information, and how to acquire it. This level requires both internal and external "work." Some information is internal; you'll seek it via a process of self-assessment.

•Step 3: Examine the alternativesAs you gather knowledge, you will probably find numerous viable pathways of action, or options. You may also use your creativity and other facts to design new possibilities. At this stage, you will identify all conceivable and desired choices.

•Step 4: Evaluate the evidenceDraw on your facts and emotions to envision what it would be like if you carried out each of the possibilities to their conclusion. Evaluate whether the requirement specified in Step 1 would be addressed or resolved via the adoption of each alternative. As you go through this arduous internal process, you'll begin to prefer specific alternatives that appear to have a better probability of accomplishing your objective. Finally, rank the options in a priority order, depending upon your personal value system.

•Step 5: Select from the available optionsOnce you have examined all the data, you are ready to pick the option that appears to be the best one for you. You may even select a mix of possibilities. Your option in Step 5 may very likely be the same or similar to the alternative you selected at the top of your list at the conclusion of Step 4.

•Step 6: Do something.You're now ready to take some good action by starting to execute the option you picked in Step 5.

•Step 7: Review your choice & its repercussionsIn this last step, analyze the effects of your choice and evaluate whether or not it has addressed the need you stated in Step 1.

If the choice has not addressed the specified need, you may choose to redo some parts of the process to arrive at a new decision.

Chapter 3

Assessing Physical Damage And Understanding The Importance Of Exercise

The typical lifespan is 80 years, give or take a few years. The reality is that a large proportion of individuals look and feel 80 before their time.

They have:

• saggy, dry skin, unattractive posture, an uneven and unsteady step, hurting joints.Imagine what their interior machinery is like if their outward appearance is so bad.

Most likely, it's much worse:

Heart problems, excess sugar and fat in or around vital organs conditions such as diabetes, mental stress, high blood pressure, and cardiovascular disease that are quietly festering.

If fitness officials had it their way, they'd design laws to make exercise necessary as soon as a newborn leaves the cradle, not during the adolescent years when obesity is prone to occur.

But fitness shouldn't be connected to any age. You may start at 10 or at 30—even at 50 or 60. Fitness should not be considered as the solution to an ailment you already have, but as preventive maintenance.

Start with the inquiry, "How do I look?" Do any of these responses apply to you?

 Am I overweight? Do I look like an apple or a pear? Do I have a spare tire? Has my skin gotten abnormally dry, nearly paper-thin? Next, ask: "How do I feel?"

Do my joints suffer before or after any physical exertion?

If fitness officials had it their way, they'd design laws to make exercise necessary as soon as a newborn leaves the cradle, not during the adolescent years when obesity is prone to occur.

But fitness shouldn't be connected with any age restriction. You may start at 10 or at 30. even at the ages of 50 and 60?The idea is that fitness should not be viewed as a cure for a disease that has already developed.As the adage goes, don't wait for disease to hit.

Start with the question, how? How do I look? Do any of these responses relate to you?

Am I overweight, appearing like an apple or pear?

Do I have a spare tire around my waist?

Has my skin gotten abnormally dry, nearly paper-thin?

Next, ask:

How do I feel?

Do my joints suffer before or after any physical exertion?

Am I continually concerned and anxious?

Do I feel sleepy and sluggish most of the time?

Do I suffer from mood swings?

Last question,

How am I doing?

Is walking and climbing stairs difficult?

Do I have trouble concentrating?

Is running impossible for me now?

Do I Find it difficult to sit upright, preferring to slouch or crook my shoulders?

You've finished your basic evaluation. Note, however, that different exercise or fitness experts will have their own measures or indices for analyzing your body's general status, and one isn't better than the other.

As long as they embrace all facets of the person ? physical, psychological,psychological, and mental ? TheyThey are as legitimate as the next person's evaluation charts.

Turning You into a Fitness Buff!

After going through the assessment phase, you're probably experiencing what some people fondly call a ""rude awakening."."

If you're not psychologically prepared to embrace exercise, please don't push yourself. Just be acquainted with its advantages, and when you're genuinely oriented towards giving it a crack in the can, move gently.gently.

Chapter 4

Optimize Your Bedtime Fervently.

Taking control of your daily sleep schedule is a powerful step toward getting better sleep. To start leveraging your calendar to your advantage, consider applying these four strategies:

Set a Fixed Wake-Up Time:

It's near to impossible for your body to grow accustomed to a healthy sleep habit if you're continuously waking up at various times. Pick a wake-up time and stick with it, even on weekends or other days when you would otherwise be tempted to sleep in. Schedule Sleep

Time:If you want to make sure that you're receiving the necessary amount of sleep each night, then you need to designate that time in your calendar. Considering your predetermined wake-up time, proceed backwards and select a desired bedtime. Whenever possible, give yourself extra time before bed to get ready for sleep. Be Careful With Naps: To sleep better at night, it's necessary to exercise prudence with naps. If you nap for too long or too late in the day, it might throw off your sleep cycle and make it difficult to go to sleep when you want to.

The optimal time to sleep is just after lunch in the early afternoon, and the best nap duration is roughly 20 minutes.

Adjust Your Schedule Gradually:

When you need to modify your sleep pattern, it's preferable to make modifications little-by-little and over time, with a maximum variation of 1-2 hours each night. This helps your body to become accustomed to the changes so that following your new routine is more sustainable.

Chapter 5

Maintain Friendly Relationships

Strong connections and remaining in touch with friends and loved ones may enhance mental wellness.

For one, the risk of depression is increased among people with low-quality relationships. Those with the worst quality social interactions had more than twice the risk of depression compared to people with the greatest quality connections.

Similarly, feeling lonely is connected with an increased likelihood of poor self-rated health and depression. It is also associated with numerous health concerns, such as headaches, palpitations, and lower back, neck, or shoulder discomfort.

Even if you cannot get together with friends or family in person, set a time to catch up via phone or video conversation once a week. Or, just start conversing with a neighbor when you see them.